Ebook Title
Discover The Proven Methods To Eliminate Pancreatitis With This Superb Meal Plans In 30 Days

Copyright Page:

The author retains full copyright rights to this publication at all times. The author has made every reasonable effort to ensure that this publication is free from error. However, the author assumes no responsibility (legal or otherwise) for any errors, omissions, or alternate interpretations of the subject matter contained herein.

This publication is purely an information product. It is not intended for use as a source of legal, accounting or other forms of authoritative advice. No guarantees of income, sales, or results are claimed or implied. Figures and statistics are true only for the author and are given for example purposes only.

- Chapter 1 13
- What Is Pancreatitis: 13
  - The pancreas has two leading roles in the body 14
  - Kinds of Pancreatitis 15
  - • Acute pancreatitis 15
  - Chronic pancreatitis 15
- Chapter 2 18
- What are the symptoms of pancreatitis? 18
  - Other common symptoms 18
  - What Causes Pancreatitis? 19
  - Situations that could lead to pancreatitis consist 22
- Chapter3 24
- Risk factors For Pancreatitis: 24
  - Extreme alcohol intake 24
  - Cigarette smoking 24
  - Obesity. 24
  - Family history of pancreatitis. 25
  - Pseudocyst. 25
  - Infection 25
  - Kidney failure 25
  - Breathing difficulties 26
  - Pancreatic cancer 26
  - What Are Other Causes of Pancreatitis 27
- CHAPTER 4 29

Which Drugs Cause Pancreatitis? 29
What Are the Other Symptoms of Pancreatitis? 30
Treatment & Management of pancreatitis: 33
Chapter 5 36
Prevention of pancreatitis: 36
How Is Pancreatitis Detected? 36
Blood tests: 38
Imaging studies 39
- How Common Is Pancreatitis 40
How Does Pancreatitis Develop? 41
Chapter 6 44
What Is a Pancreatic Cyst? 44
What is the pancreatitis prognosis 45
Pancreatic function test: 45
What is the treatment for pancreatitis? 46
. ...46
Surgery 48
Chapter 7 49
Pancreatitis diet: 49
Pancreatitis home remedies: 50
Lifestyle changes 50
Alternative techniques for pain control 51
Pancreatitis pain 51
What to eat if you have pancreatitis: 52

Pancreatitis recovery diet: 55
Diet tips: 55
Can pancreatitis be stopped? 57
Medications for pancreatitis: 58
Is there a diet for pancreatitis? 58
NUTRITION FOR CHRONIC PANCREATITIS: 59
CAUSES OF DYSPEPSIA 59
Chapter 8 61
What Is Necrotizing Pancreatitis and Exactly How Is It Treated? 61
   Is this cause for concern? 61
   What causes necrotizing pancreatitis to develop? ...62
   What are the symptoms 63
   Other common symptoms 63
   How is it detected? 64
   What treatment opportunities are accessible? 65
Chapter 9 67
Alternative Medicine Treatments For Chronic Pancreatitis: 67
Chapter10 78
Natural Remedies for Pancreatitis Relief 78
   Pancreatitis and Your Diet: 79
   Healthy Foods to Eat With Chronic Pancreatitis: 81
   Pancreatitis and Weight Loss 81

Remedies for Pancreatitis Relief 81
Antioxidants 82
Glutamine: 83
Omega-3 Fatty Acids 83
Should You Use Natural Remedies for Pancreatitis Relief? 84
Natural Relief from Pancreatitis Pain 85
Pancreatic Pain Relief the Natural Way: 86
Alternative Physical Therapies for Pancreatitis 88
Chapter 11 90
Pancreatitis Diet: 90
CHRONIC PANCREATITIS PAIN MANAGEMENT AND TREATMENT 91
Pain Management 91
Restricted Role of Endoscopic Retrograde Cholangiopancreatography (ERCP) 92
Surgery: 92
Whipple Procedure: 93
TPIAT: 93
Antioxidant therapies: 94
Bilateral Thoracoscopic Splanchnicectomy: 95
The following treatments are usually suggested for chronic pancreatitis. 95
Lifestyle changes 95
Endoscopic surgery 96

The Frey procedure 97
Autologous pancreatic islet cell transplantation (APICT) 97
Chapter12 99
7-Day Pancreatitis Diet Meal Plan 99
Pancreatitis Diet Foods to Eat 100
Pancreatitis Diet Foods to Shun 101
Organ meats 101
Fried foods 101
Treated meats 101
Drinks with added sugar 102
Full-fat dairy 102
High-fat spreads 102
Selecting a Pancreatitis Diet: 102
Pancreatitis Diet Meal Plan 104
Pancreatitis Diet Sample Menu 104
Monday 104
Tuesday 105
Wednesday 105
Thursday 105
Friday 105
Saturday 106
Sunday 106
· Day 1: Monday 106

Breakfast: Banana Yogurt Pots 107

Nutrition 107

Day 2: Tuesday 109

Breakfast: Tomato and Watermelon Salad 109

Day 3: Wednesday 112

Breakfast: Blueberry Oats Dish 112

Nutrition 112

Day 4: Thursday 114

Breakfast: Banana Yogurt Vessels 114

Lunch: Blend Bean Salad 115

Day 5: Friday 117

Breakfast: Tomato and Watermelon Salad 117

Lunch: Panzanella Salad 117

Day 6: Saturday 119

Breakfast: Blueberry Oats Bowl 119

Lunch: Quinoa and Blend Fried Veg 119

Day 7: Sunday 122

Breakfast: Banana Yogurt Pots 122

Lunch: Moroccan Chickpea Broth 122

Nutrition 122

Pancreatitis Diet Shopping List 124

Introduction:

Pancreatitis is irritation in the pancreas. The pancreas is an extended, flat gland that sits placed behind the stomach in the upper abdomen. The pancreas makes enzymes that aid digestion and hormones that assist to

regulate the way your body processes sugar (glucose).

Pancreatitis could happen as acute pancreatitis — denoting it shows unexpectedly and lasts for days. Or pancreatitis could show as chronic pancreatitis, which is pancreatitis that happens over several years.

Mild cases of pancreatitis might heal devoid of treatment, though serious cases could cause life-threatening problems.

- Pancreatitis is an inflammation of the pancreas. Of the several causes of

pancreatitis, the most usual are alcohol intake and gallstones.
- About 210,000 cases of acute pancreatitis occur in the U.S. every year.

Chapter 1
What Is Pancreatitis:

Pancreatitis is mainly inflammation in the pancreas. The pancreas is a lengthy, flat gland that sits placed behind the stomach in the upper abdomen. The pancreas yield enzymes that aid digestion and hormones that assist in regulating the mode your body processes sugar (glucose).

Pancreatitis is genuinely a disease in which your pancreas becomes swollen. The pancreas is a large gland at the back of your stomach and next to your small intestine. Your pancreas does two essentials things:
- It releases potent digestive enzymes into your small intestine to assist you digest food.

- It discharges insulin and glucagon into your bloodstream. These hormones support your body to regulate how it uses food for energy.

Your pancreas could be hurt when digestive enzymes start working before your pancreas discharges them.

Pancreatitis is a swelling of the pancreas, a gland that sits at the back of the stomach and near the first segment of the small intestine, the duodenum.

The pancreas has two leading roles in the body:

· It secretes digestive enzymes to aid the intestines to digest food.
· It assists in regulating blood sugar levels by manufacturing insulin and glucagon.
Pancreatitis comes about whenever the pancreas's enzymes begin digesting pancreatic tissues.

This could lead to swelling, bleeding, and harm to the pancreas. Gallstones,

Alcoholism, and specific types of medication could cause pancreatitis.

There are two leading forms of pancreatitis: acute and chronic. "Pancreatitis" is frequently used synonymously with "acute pancreatitis," since this form of the disease appears.

Kinds of Pancreatitis:

The two types of pancreatitis are acute and chronic.

- **Acute pancreatitis** is caused by unexpected inflammation that goes on for a short time. It could go from mild discomfort to a severe and life-threatening illness. Most individuals with acute pancreatitis recover fully after getting the correct treatment. In severe cases, acute pancreatitis could lead to bleeding, severe tissue damage, infection, and cysts. Acute pancreatitis can also damage other essential organs like the heart, lungs, and kidneys.

- **Chronic pancreatitis** is long-lasting inflammation. It most regularly occurs after an incidence of acute pancreatitis. Another major cause is the intake of alcohol for an extended period. Injury to your pancreas from heavy alcohol use might not cause symptoms for several years; however, then you might unexpectedly have severe pancreatitis symptoms.

Pancreatitis could happen as acute pancreatitis — meaning it appears suddenly and lasts for days. Or pancreatitis could also occur as chronic pancreatitis, which is pancreatitis that arises over several years.

Mild cases of pancreatitis might go away without treatment; though severe cases could cause life-threatening problems.
Chronic pancreatitis arises when the pancreas becomes more dented and less effective over time, typically because of alcohol abuse.

It's been projected that more than half of chronic pancreatitis cases can be ascribed to Alcoholism, and the lengthier the history of drinking, the higher the likely damage.

Chronic pancreatitis might also be triggered by infection, medication, or a family history of the disease.

Persons with chronic pancreatitis always have had numerous bouts of acute pancreatitis. The pain in the abdomen that accompanies acute pancreatitis might still be present, though not as strong.

Owning to the long-term harm sustained by the pancreas, chronic pancreatitis may also lead to diabetes owing to weakened insulin secretion, as well as difficulty digesting and absorbing the nutrients necessary to keep your body running as it should be.

Chapter 2

What are the symptoms of pancreatitis?

Abdominal pain is one of the significant symptoms of necrotizing pancreatitis. It could build slowly or come on swiftly. Severe pain could be felt in front, very close to your stomach, and also wrap around your back. The pain might last for some days.

The pain may also become worse after eating, and your abdomen might become enflamed.

Other common symptoms comprise:
- fever
- nausea
- vomiting
- dryness
- rapid heart rate

What Causes Pancreatitis?

Pancreatitis happens when digestive enzymes become triggered while still in the pancreas, irritating your pancreas' cells and causing swelling.

With recurring bouts of acute pancreatitis, harm to the pancreas can happen and lead to chronic pancreatitis. Scar tissue might develop in the pancreas, causing loss of function. A poorly working pancreas could cause digestion complications and diabetes.

The most common causes of acute pancreatitis are gallstones and alcohol.
Gallstones are pebble-like deposits that form in the gallbladder due to the hardening of two elements: cholesterol and bilirubin.

Bilirubin is a byproduct of the breaking down of red blood cells found in bile (this substance also contributes.
The most common causes of acute pancreatitis are gallstones and alcohol.

Gallstones are pebble-like deposits that form in the gallbladder due to the hardening of two substances: cholesterol and bilirubin. Bilirubin is a

Result of the breaking down of red blood cells found in bile (this substance also contributes to jaundice).

Research shows that gallstones cause 42 to 72 percent of acute pancreatitis cases, according to the American College of Gastroenterology.

Small gallstones — typically less than 5 millimeters — heighten the risk of pancreatitis.

It's believed that gallstones cause pancreatitis by crafting an obstruction in the pancreatic duct. This pushes digestive enzymes back into the pancreas, which causes inflammation.

According to the American College of Gastroenterology, the second most common cause of acute pancreatitis is alcohol intake, which accounts for at least 27 percent of cases.

It's uncertain just how alcohol causes the condition, though it's understood that the way the pancreas processes alcohol may produce toxic compounds to the organ's acinar cells.

Alcohol could also alert acinar cells to the consequence of cholecystokinin, a hormone-free by the duodenum that stimulates the discharge of digestive enzymes.
It's tough to say just how many drinks would lead to acute pancreatitis.

One research, which tracked Swedish men and women for numerous years and was distributed in the *British Journal of Surgery*, establish that the risk of acute pancreatitis increased 53 percent with every increment of six drinks consumed on one occasion.

It's worth noting that the National Institute on Alcohol Abuse and Alcoholism describes binge drinking as five drinks in about two hours for women, and six drinks in about two hours for men. The Substance Abuse and Mental Health Services Administration describes heavy drinking as binge drinking for six or more days in a month.

Pancreatitis happens when digestive enzymes become triggered while still in the pancreas, irritating your pancreas' cells and bringing about inflammation.

With frequent bouts of acute pancreatitis, harm to the pancreas can arise and lead to chronic pancreatitis. Scar tissue might form in the pancreas, causing loss of function. A poorly working pancreas could cause digestion complications and diabetes.

Situations that could lead to pancreatitis consist of:
· Abdominal surgery
· Alcoholism
· Certain medications
· Cystic fibrosis
· Gallstones
· Extraordinary calcium levels in the blood (hypercalcemia), which could be

caused by an intense parathyroid gland (hyperparathyroidism)
· Extraordinary triglyceride levels in the blood (hypertriglyceridemia)

- Infection
- Destruction to the abdomen
- Obesity
- Pancreatic cancer

Endoscopic retrograde cholangiopancreatography (ERCP) is a process used to treat gallstones and could lead to pancreatitis.

At times, a cause for pancreatitis is never found.

Chapter 3

Risk factors For Pancreatitis:

Elements that push up your risk of pancreatitis consist of:

Extreme alcohol intake. Studies demonstrate that substantial alcohol consumers (folks who consume five to six drinks a day) are at a more significant risk of pancreatitis.

Cigarette smoking. Cigarette smokers are usually three times more likely to have chronic pancreatitis, as compared with nonsmokers. The good news is leaving smoking to lessen your risk by about half

Obesity. You're more likely to have pancreatitis if you're obese.

Family history of pancreatitis.

The role of genetics is becoming more and more known in chronic pancreatitis. If you have family members with the condition, your odds increase — particularly when combined with other risk factors.
Problems
Pancreatitis can cause grave complications, comprising:

Pseudocyst. Acute pancreatitis could cause fluid and debris to gather in cyst like pockets in your pancreas. A huge pseudocyst that ruptures can cause problems like internal bleeding and Infection.

Infection. Acute pancreatitis can make your pancreas susceptible to bacteria and Infection. Pancreatic infections are severe and need intensive treatment, such as surgery, to eliminate the infected tissue.

Kidney failure. Acute pancreatitis might cause kidney failure, which could be treated with dialysis if kidney failure is severe and persistent.

Breathing difficulties. Acute pancreatitis can cause chemical alterations in your body that affect your lung function, making your blood's oxygen level fall to seriously low levels.

- **Diabetes.** Harm to insulin-producing cells in your pancreas from chronic pancreatitis could lead to diabetes, a disease that affects the manner your body uses blood sugar.
- **Malnutrition.** Both acute and chronic pancreatitis can make your pancreas create fewer enzymes necessary to break down and process nutrients from the food you consume. This could lead to malnutrition, diarrhea, and weight loss, although you might be consuming the same food or quantity.

Pancreatic cancer. Long-standing inflammation in your pancreas triggered by chronic pancreatitis is a risk factor for developing pancreatic cancer.

In usual conditions, digestive enzymes are found in cells in an inactive state.

Conversely, under the influence of various factors can occur, triggering them, and they start to digest the parenchyma of the pancreas and its tissue as only as exogenous food.

Inflammation of the pancreas and the discharge of digestive enzymes into the blood causes the development of severe intoxication. Differentiate acute and chronic pancreatitis.

The significant change is that acute pancreatitis may reestablish the normal function of the pancreas; the chronic form over time witnessed a steady weakening incapacity.

What Are Other Causes of Pancreatitis?

Medical students use the mnemonic "I GET SMASHED" to recall the following added causes of pancreatitis:
· **I**diopathic (unknown causes)

- **G**allstones
- **E**thanol (alcohol)
- **S**hock
- **S**teroids
- **M**umps, as well as other infections, like Ascaris, lumbricoides parasites, Coxsackie B virus, viral hepatitis, leptospirosis, and HIV, and **m**alignancy (tumors)
- **A**utoimmune pancreatitis, which grows from a surplus of IgG4 antibodies
- **S**corpion stings
- **H**yperlipidemia and **h**ypertriglyceridemia (raised levels of fat in your blood)

and **h**ypercalcemia (elevated blood calcium levels) which might cause calcium to

deposit in the pancreatic duct or facilitate the initiation of pancreatic enzymes)

- ERCP, or endoscopic retrograde cholangiopancreatography, an aggressive diagnostic procedure

- **D**rugs

CHAPTER 4
Which Drugs Cause Pancreatitis?

Drugs cause pancreatitis in numerous ways. For instance, they may be toxic to the pancreas, tighten the pancreatic duct, cause vascular problems, or affect the pancreatic handling systems.

Drug-induced pancreatitis is uncommon. It's projected that medication is only accountable for 1.4 percent to 2 percent of cases. However, many different drugs can cause it.

According to an article widely circulated in the journal *Baylor University Medical Center Proceedings,*
there are published case reports of drug-induced pancreatitis for more than 42 of the top 200 most recommended drugs.

The report notes the six most typical drugs or drug classes that cause pancreatitis:

Statins, which lower cholesterol and comprise simvastatin (Zocor) and atorvastatin (Lipitor)

ACE inhibitors, which contain enalapril (Vasotec) and lisinopril (Zestril), for hypertension and congestive heart failure
Estrogens in oral contraception and hormone replacement remedy
Diuretics, comprising furosemide (Lasix) and hydrochlorothiazide (Microzide)
Exceptionally active antiretroviral therapy (HAART), containing lamivudine (Epivir) and nelfinavir (Viracept) for HIV
 Valproic acid (Depakote, Depacon, Stavzor) for seizures

What Are the Other Symptoms of Pancreatitis?

Signs and symptoms of pancreatitis might differ, reliant on which type you experience. Acute pancreatitis signs and symptoms contain:
· Upper abdominal discomfort

- Abdominal pain that transmits to your back
- Abdominal pain that becomes worse after eating
- Fever
- Speedy pulse
- Nausea
- Unsettled stomach
- Gentleness while touching the abdomen

Chronic pancreatitis signs and symptoms include:
- Upper abdominal discomfort
- Losing weight short of trying
- Oily, stinking stools (steatorrhea)

Symptoms of acute pancreatitis
- Fever
- Higher heart rate
- Nausea and vomiting
- Swollen and tender belly
- Discomfort in the upper part of your belly that goes straight into your back. Eating could make it worse, particularly foods high in fat.

Symptoms of chronic pancreatitis:

The symptoms of chronic pancreatitis are related to those of acute pancreatitis. However, you may also have:

- Frequent pain in your upper belly that goes to your back. This pain may be disabling.
- <u>Diarrhea</u> and weight loss since your pancreas isn't discharging sufficient enzymes to break down food.
- Troubled stomach and vomiting

When to see a physician
Try to book an appointment with your doctor if you have constant abdominal pain.

Get instant medical assistance if your abdominal pain is so severe that you can't sit

still or find a place that makes you more relaxed.

There are two types of pancreatitis — acute and chronic — and their symptoms vary. Acute pancreatitis comes on unexpectedly and typically subsides within a week with treatment, though severe cases could go on longer.

It's most habitually caused by gallstones or too much alcohol; however, certain drugs or elevated triglycerides can bring about an attack. The primary symptom of acute pancreatitis is a sharp, unexpected pain in the abdomen that you may also sense in your back. Other symptoms consist of Fever and vomiting.

Chronic pancreatitis is most commonly the result of Alcoholism, and it also involves pain in the abdomen that radiates in your back and may deteriorate after eating — though, sometimes, there is no pain at all. Other symptoms of chronic pancreatitis might contain greasy, light-colored stools, and weight loss.

Treatment & Management of pancreatitis:

The manifestation of acute pancreatitis or acute deteriorations of chronic needs urgent hospitalization in the surgical department of a hospital: however, a small delay can have serious consequences.

Hence, in the case of you or your family described signs, you should instantly call an ambulance.

In the period of reduction of chronic pancreatitis, it is suggested to give up alcohol and to stick to a proper diet.

Patients show a diet with reduced fat and improved protein content (meat, fish, and cheese) are left out, spicy food, and crude fiber (cabbage, raw apples, oranges).

Pancreatitis Treatment clinic for the diagnosis of examination, which comprises General clinical examination of blood, which is carried out within order to identify signs of inflammation (rise in the number of leukocytes, improved erythrocyte sedimentation rate, etc.);

A biochemical blood test to identify high levels of pancreatic enzymes (amylase, lipase, trypsin); urinalysis discovery of amylase in urine also point to pancreatitis;

Ultrasound analysis of abdominal cavity allows to notice changes in the pancreas and other organs (for instance, gall bladder); gastroscopy (endoscopy); roentgenography of organs of an abdominal cavity; endoscopic retrograde cholangiopancreatography (ERCP); fecal; functional tests.

· In acute pancreatitis, employ a starvation diet, analgesics for relief of pain, drip intravenous saline or colloid solutions, inhibitors of proteolytic enzymes (drugs that block the activity of enzymes and other drugs. In unusual cases, you might require surgical treatment.

Management of chronic pancreatitis comprises diet, analgesics, vitamins, replacement therapy enzymes, the treatment of diabetes and other endocrine disorders, initial treatment of gallstone disease.

Chapter 5

Prevention of pancreatitis:

Prevention of the disease consists of total abstinence from alcohol, appropriate treatment of diseases of the biliary tract, stomach and duodenum, suitable diet (with the exclusion of coarse animal fats and hot spices).

In chronic pancreatitis, these activities will hamper the development of exacerbations.

How Is Pancreatitis Detected?

You'll have a physical examination, and your physician will order blood tests and imaging tests to sanction whether you have either acute or severe pancreatitis.

All through the physical examination, your doctor might feel your stomach to see whether your muscles are very rigid or your abdomen is tender.

The blood test, which could only point to pancreatitis — not diagnose it for sure — measures the amount of two digestive enzymes in the pancreas.

With the commencement of acute pancreatitis, the levels of those enzymes are higher than average — usually more than three times the standard level, according to the National Institutes of Health. Other blood tests might measure kidney function and white blood cell count.

Your doctor might also order the following imaging tests to check for the manifestation of gallstones, inflammation, and other changes:

· X-rays
· Ultrasounds
· Computerized tomography (CT) scans
· Endoscopic ultrasounds (EUS)

- Magnetic resonance cholangiopancreatography (MRCP)
- The EUS test contains putting a lighted tube into your mouth and down into your intestine to check for obstruction or damage.

- The MRCP is a type of MRI in which you are injected with a dye that irradiates the pancreas and neighboring areas.

- Chronic pancreatitis is diagnosed in the same manner. The physician might go for various blood tests because, in chronic pancreatitis, the digestive enzyme levels might look normal.

Stool tests are standard, ever since chronic pancreatitis compromises the organ's ability to digest and absorb nutrients, which yields changes in the stool.

There are some tests that alone, or in combination, will help establish the diagnosis of pancreatitis.

Blood tests:

Amylase and lipase levels are usually raised in cases of acute pancreatitis. These blood tests might not be raised in cases of chronic pancreatitis.

These are typically the first tests to establish the diagnosis of pancreatitis, as these results are usually readily accessible. Other blood tests may be ordered, for instance:

- **Liver** and kidney function tests
- Tests for Infection
- Tests for **anemia**

Imaging studies:

A CT (computed tomography) scan of the abdomen might be ordered to picture the pancreas, appraise the extent of inflammation, and any of the likely complications that can arise from pancreatitis, like bleeding or pseudocyst (a collection of fluid) formation. The **CT scan** may also identify gallstones (a leading cause of pancreatitis) and other deformities of the biliary system.

Ultrasound imaging can be used to see gallstones and defects of the biliary system.

Since ultrasound imaging does not produce radiation, this modality is often the initial imaging test gotten in cases of pancreatitis.

Relying on the fundamental cause of pancreatitis and the severity of illness, further testing may be ordered.

- **How Common Is Pancreatitis?**

Pancreatitis is the cause of more than 550,000 hospitalizations every year in the United States, according to the data released by the National Institute of Diabetes and Digestive and Kidney Diseases.

A publication in the *American Journal of Gastroenterology* noted that every year there are projected 6 to 76 cases of pancreatitis per every 100,000 individuals globally.

Acute pancreatitis affects men and women equally; however, men are more

susceptible to developing chronic pancreatitis.

For some persons, acute pancreatitis may need a lengthy (a week or more) hospital stay after causing grim issues such as dehydration, low blood pressure, and probably organ failure. These symptoms typically lessen in a few days.

Approximately one in five pancreatitis cases are categorized as severe. In chronic pancreatitis, the enzymes eating away at the organ lead to pancreatic necrosis or death of pancreatic tissue. Besides, pancreatic necrosis is not deadly on its own.
Severe pancreatitis could also cause organ failure, gastrointestinal bleeding, and perhaps death.

How Does Pancreatitis Develop?

In the pancreas, cells termed acinar cells produce proenzymes, which are inactive substances that turn into enzymes via metabolic processes.

These proenzymes travel to the small intestine through the pancreatic duct, where they are transformed into active forms.

Once active, the enzymes get to work processing carbohydrates, proteins, fats, and

other food substances.

However, if the acinar cells become spoiled or the pancreatic duct is battered or blocked, the proenzymes may add up in the pancreas and activate hastily.

When this occurs, the enzymes digest cell membranes in the pancreas, generating an inflammatory reaction from the immune system.

The most common causes of acute pancreatitis are gallstones and alcohol.
Gallstones are pebble-like deposits accumulated in the gallbladder due to the hardening of two constituents:

cholesterol and bilirubin. Bilirubin is a result of the breaking down of red blood cells that are gotten in bile (this substance also contributes.

Chapter 6

What Is a Pancreatic Cyst?

A pancreatic cyst is a pocket of fluid living on or in the pancreas. These cysts, which might be caused by pancreatitis though sometimes appear on their own, can be benign or cancerous. Warning signs, when there are any, consist of abdominal pain, abdominal swelling, and vomiting.

However, since these cysts don't typically cause pain, they're usually found through CT and MRI scans that have been recommended for purposes other than probing the pancreas.

Pancreatic cysts are regularly nonthreatening and go away on their own, though, if left untreated, some may lead to cancer. Surgery is used to get rid of both benign and cancerous cysts.

What is the pancreatitis prognosis?

Pancreatitis can range from a mild, self-limited disease to a situation with life-threatening problems.

Pancreatic function test:

The pancreatic function test, also termed the secretin stimulation test, shows whether your pancreas is usually responding to secretin. Secretin is a hormone that causes your pancreas to discharge a fluid that assists in digesting food.

During the test, your physician will run a tube through your nose or throat and down into your small intestine. They'll inject secretin into your vein, then take samples of fluid via the tube.

Your doctor will send the liquid to a lab to help diagnose pancreatitis or other conditions that upset your pancreas.

What is the treatment for pancreatitis?

.

In many cases of acute pancreatitis, admission to the hospital is required, though some chronic pancreatitis can be managed in an outpatient setting.

Depending on the original cause of pancreatitis, Management may differ to address the definite cause. In general, though, the following treatment regimen will often be introduced for the treatment of pancreatitis.

First-line treatment will consist of:

- Fasting to assist the pancreas in resting and recuperating.
- IV fluids to stop **dehydration** while fasting

- Pancreatitis can be very disturbing; thus, intravenous pain medication is always necessary.
-

If pancreatitis is due to an obstructing gallstone, surgical intervention may be needed to eliminate the gallstone and get rid of the gallbladder. Intervention may also be necessary to treat a pseudocyst or to take out part of the affected pancreas.

If alcohol ingestion is the cause of pancreatitis, abstinence from alcohol and an alcohol rehabilitation program will be suggested.

If a medication or chemical exposure is known to be the cause of pancreatitis, then eliminating the medication or offending exposure is prescribed.

If high **triglycerides** are the primary cause of pancreatitis, then your health-care professional may propose medication to reduce the patient's **triglyceride levels**.

Treatment for acute or chronic pancreatitis often consists of hospitalization. The pancreas is a strategic provider to your digestive processes and needs to rest to set right.

Thus, you may receive specially tailored fluids and nutrition intravenously (IV) or through a tube that goes from your nose directly into your stomach. This is termed a nasogastric feeding tube.

Medication may help control the pain. You may also get artificial digestive enzymes for chronic pancreatitis if your pancreas isn't manufacturing enough of them on its own.

They are restarting an oral diet hinge on your condition. Some folks feel better after a couple of days. Other individuals need a week or two to heal sufficiently.

Surgery

You may require surgery if other treatments aren't working. If your doctor detects gallstones, surgery to eliminate the gallbladder may help. Surgery can also get rid of diseased parts of your pancreas.

Chapter 7

Pancreatitis diet:

A low-fat, healthy diet plays a significant role in recuperating from pancreatitis. Individuals with chronic pancreatitis, in particular, need to be cautious about the amount of fat they eat, since their pancreas function has become compromised. Try to limit or shun the following foods:
- Red meat
- fried food
- full-fat dairy
- sugary desserts
- sweetened beverages
- caffeine
- alcohol

Eat small meals all through the day to put less stress on your digestive system. Stick to foods that are very high in protein and antioxidants, and drink lots of fluids to stay hydrated.

Your doctor might also give you vitamin supplements to guarantee that you're getting the nutrients you genuinely need.

Pancreatitis home remedies:

It's vital to see your doctor if you feel you have pancreatitis, particularly if you have persistent pain in your abdomen. There are steps you could take at home to complement your treatment and help avoid pancreatitis.

Lifestyle changes:

Stop smoking tobacco and control drinking alcohol in excess to help you heal more swiftly and totally. Discuss these issues with your doctor if you need assistance.

Sustaining a healthy weight can help you circumvent gallstones, a significant cause of pancreatitis. Eating a balanced diet and staying hydrated can also help you recuperate from and avert pancreatitis.

Alternative techniques for pain control

You'll possibly be given IV pain medication in the hospital. Alternative therapies may also help lessen pancreatitis pain.
You can try yoga, relaxation exercises like deep breathing, and meditation if orthodox treatments don't lessen your pain.

These alternative treatments emphasize slow, measured movements that can take your mind off your uneasiness.

A 2019 study found that acupuncture may offer short-term pain relief for folks with chronic pancreatitis. Even though more studies are required, some studies have also recommended that taking antioxidant supplements may help relieve pain from pancreatitis.

Pancreatitis pain

Pain-related with pancreatitis may last from a few minutes to many hours at a time. In severe cases, uneasiness from chronic pancreatitis could become persistent.

Your pain is projected to increase after you eat or when you're lying down. Try sitting up or leaning forward to make yourself more satisfied.

Activities like yoga, meditation, and acupuncture may assist with pain from pancreatitis. You could also try taking pain medication or antioxidant supplements to help get rid of the pain.

Surgery is presently the last resort for treating pancreatitis, though, research from 2019 showed that undergoing surgery earlier in the course of treatment may help with pain relief.

What to eat if you have pancreatitis:

To get your pancreas in good physical shape, concentrate on foods rich in protein, low in animal fats, and antioxidants. Go for lean meats, beans and lentils, clear soups, and dairy replacements (like flax milk and almond milk).

Your pancreas won't have to work as hard to process these.

Research states that some individuals with pancreatitis can bear up to 30 to 40% of calories from fat when it's from whole-food plant sources or medium-chain triglycerides (MCTs).

Others do better with much lower fat consumption, like 50 grams or less per day.
Spinach, blueberries, cherries, and whole grains can help safeguard your digestion and fight the free radicals that harm your organs.

If you're looking for something sweet, reach for fruit in
place of added sugars since those with pancreatitis are at high risk for diabetes.
Ponder cherry tomatoes, cucumbers and hummus, and fruit as your go-to snacks.
Your pancreas will thank you.

What not to eat if you have pancreatitis
Foods to limit comprise:
- red meat
- organ meats
- fried foods
- deep-fries and potato chips
- mayonnaise
- margarine and butter
- full-fat dairy
-
- pastries and desserts with additional sugars
- beverages with added sugars

If you're trying to fight pancreatitis, shun trans-fatty acids in your diet.
Fried or heavily processed foods, such as French fries and fast-food hamburgers, are some of the worst offenders. Organ meats, full-fat dairy, potato chips, and mayonnaise also top the list of foods to go away from.

Cooked or deep-fried foods might prompt a flare-up of pancreatitis. You'll also need to cut back on the refined flour found in cakes, pastries, and cookies. These foods can tax the digestive system by making your insulin levels to rise.

Pancreatitis recovery diet:

If you're recuperating from acute or chronic pancreatitis, shun drinking alcohol. If you smoke, you'll also need to leave it. Concentrate on eating a low-fat diet that won't tax or exacerbate your pancreas.

You should also stay well hydrated. Have an electrolyte beverage or a bottle of water every time.

If you've been hospitalized owing to a pancreatitis flare-up, your doctor will maybe refer you to a dietitian to aid you in studying how to change your eating habits always.

Persons with chronic pancreatitis always experience malnutrition owing to their reduced pancreas function. Vitamins A, D, E, and K are usually found to be deficient as a consequence of pancreatitis.

Diet tips:

Continuously consult with your doctor or dietician before modifying your eating habits when you have pancreatitis. These are some tips they might propose:

- Eat between six and eight small meals all through the day to help recuperate from pancreatitis. This is easier on your digestive system than consuming two or three large meals.

- Use MCTs as your primary fat ever since this type of fat does not need pancreatic enzymes to be digested. MCTs can be gotten from coconut oil and palm kernel oil and is accessible at most health food stores.

- Shun overeating fiber at once, as this can slow digestion and lead to less-than-ideal absorption of nutrients from food. Fiber could also give your restricted amount of enzymes less effective.

- Take a multivitamin supplement to guarantee that you're getting the nutrition you require. You can find a vast collection of multivitamins in many stores.

Can pancreatitis be stopped?

- Some lifestyle changes can decrease the probabilities of someone getting pancreatitis, like alcohol and **smoking cessation**.
- Consuming a low-fat **diet**, and sustaining a healthy weight can lessen the risk of developing gallstones, a leading cause of pancreatitis.

The prognosis for pancreatitis centers on several factors, such as the underlying situation causing pancreatitis, the severity of pancreatitis, and the patient's age and underlying medical problems.

Patients suffering from pancreatitis can experience everything from a short self-limited illness with a full recovery to a severe course of illness that can accumulate in life-threatening complications and death.

If an individual has persistent episodes of acute pancreatitis, they may witness chronic pancreatitis, a lifelong situation that can lead to a reduced quality of life.

Medications for pancreatitis:

In general, the above treatment routine is the backbone of pancreatitis management.
Pain medication and medication to control Nausea may also be recommended.
In cases of chronic pancreatitis, your healthcare expert also may prescribe pancreatic enzyme **supplements** to assist the body in digesting certain nutrients.

Is there a diet for pancreatitis?

For persons with pancreatitis, low-fat meals that are high in nutrients is the suggested **diet**. Adequate fluid intake is also proposed to stop **dehydration**.

TREATMENT OF CHRONIC PANCREATITIS:

In the treatment of the effects of pancreatitis, preparations for the normalization of digestion comprising amylase, lipase, and protease may be suggested.
Which drug can assist?

NUTRITION FOR CHRONIC PANCREATITIS:

You can decrease the risk of exacerbation of chronic pancreatitis, observing the principles of a healthy diet.
How to eat with chronic pancreatitis?

CAUSES OF DYSPEPSIA

In many cases, dyspepsia is related to diseases of the digestive tract - gastritis, peptic ulcer, pancreatitis

Chapter 8

What Is Necrotizing Pancreatitis and Exactly How Is It Treated?

Is this cause for concern?

Necrotizing pancreatitis is a dangerous complication of acute pancreatitis. Acute pancreatitis is a swelling of the pancreas.

Your pancreas sits behind your stomach. One of its first jobs is to make enzymes that assist you digest food. Typically, those enzymes flow through a small opening into your small intestines.

If your pancreas becomes swollen, the enzymes can begin to leak into parts of the pancreas instead. These enzymes can sometimes kill pancreatic tissue in necrotizing pancreatitis.

The dead tissue can get infected and lead to life-threatening complications. Medication and elimination of the dead tissue are typically essential.

Continue reading to learn more about why this occurs, symptoms to watch out for, and more.

What causes necrotizing pancreatitis to develop?

Necrotizing pancreatitis occurs when acute pancreatitis is left untreated or isn't treated correctly. Most pancreatitis diagnoses occur from extreme alcohol intake and gallstones.

Pancreatitis may also result from:
- damage to the pancreas
- medication side effects
- high cholesterol
- high calcium levels in the blood
- autoimmune diseases, such as lupus
- pancreatic tumor
-

In occasional cases, necrotizing pancreatitis affects individuals with chronic pancreatitis. Chronic pancreatitis is a long-term situation, whereas acute cases are momentary episodes of inflammation.

What are the symptoms?

Abdominal pain is one of the significant symptoms of necrotizing pancreatitis. It can build slowly or come on rapidly. Severe pain can be sensed in front, very close to the stomach, and around your back. The pain may last for some days.
The pain may also become worse after eating, and your abdomen may become enflamed.

Other common symptoms consist of:
- fever
- nausea
- vomiting
- dehydration
- rapid heart rate

How is it detected?

Diagnosing necrotizing pancreatitis begins with an appraisal of your symptoms and medical history. After your doctor completes a physical examination, they may order diagnostic testing to rule out other probable causes.
Imaging tests usually include:

- abdominal ultrasound
- CT scan

They might also order blood tests that check for:
- pancreatic enzymes
- sodium
- potassium
- glucose
- cholesterol
- triglycerides

If an imaging test shows that a slice of your pancreatic tissue has expired, your doctor will want to eliminate some of the tissue for examination. To do this, your doctor will inject a fine needle into your pancreas to get a small piece of tissue. They'll test this tissue for signs infection.

What treatment opportunities are accessible?

Necrotizing pancreatitis needs a two-fold approach to treatment. Pancreatitis must be measured, and the dead tissue may need to be removed.

An acute attack of pancreatitis needs rest and fluids, always administered with an IV. Painkillers may be required. You may also require medications to control nausea and vomiting. In some cases, you may need to have nutrition given in the liquid form.

At times, this is done using a long tube that runs through your nose into your stomach.
If the tissue that was removed displays signs infection, you'll require antibiotics. You may also need to have the dead tissue eliminated.

If no infection is present, removing the dead tissue may not be necessary. Talk with your doctor about the risks and benefits of leaving the dead tissue alone versus eliminating it.

If removal is suggested, your doctor can cut the dead tissue using a catheter or endoscopic procedure. If these slightly invasive procedures aren't adequate, your doctor may propose open surgery to remove the tissue.

Any other type of procedure you've had arranged may be put off a few weeks. The initial goal is to get your pancreatitis under control.

Outlook

Necrotizing pancreatitis is treatable, but then, the risk of serious Infection is real.

It's essential to follow your doctor's recommendations to stop additional complications.

If you're pre-emptive about treatment, you'll likely live a long, healthy life after a period of necrotizing pancreatitis. Your doctor may advise lifestyle changes, such as shunning alcohol, to reduce your risk of future problems.

Chapter 9

Alternative Medicine Treatments For Chronic Pancreatitis:

Many folks work hard and run all day, metaphorically and literally. Eating lunch may mean purchasing a sandwich down the block and eating it between meetings. Others may be running around and require to eat something speedily.

Much of the consumed food today is extremely processed. These foods do not have living natural enzymes in them. Without these enzymes, the pancreas has more work to do. The body requires a definite amount of digestive enzymes to digest food properly.

The pancreas has to make more of its digestive enzymes to c compensate for the lack of natural enzymes coming in. If foods coming in do not have enzymes, then the pressure decreases on the pancreas.

With the present diet, many folks are also acidic, which means they lack potassium, magnesium, bicarbonate, zinc, cobalt, and other minerals and have low consumption of vitamins. As noted and worth reiterating, the pancreas cannot work well without this essential nutrients-remember the drooping plant image.

The modern diet is jam-packed with unnatural foods, sweeteners, chemicals, and dyes. These items are complicated to digest. The pancreas is working tirelessly to figure out what high fructose corn syrup is and how to break it down.

The pancreas is working tirelessly to figure out what high fructose corn syrup is and how to break it down.

Individuals face stress every day from several sources and formats. Incoming stress can upset the pancreas. Continuous stress can alter the hormonal and neural systems of the pancreas.

With stress coming from all directions, many persons turn to alcohol to de-stress. Regrettably, alcohol intake is the worst for the pancreas.

Several medications and drugs can lead to pancreatitis-the inflammation of the pancreas.

Everything on this list shares a commonality. Each item on this list causes the pancreas to be excessively overworked. The pancreas is not Superman, Miracle Woman, or Iron Man; it requires support.

It needs real nutrients, living digestive enzymes, and the ideal environment to do many vital jobs.

As you can infer, if the pancreas, the main digestive organ, is sick, people will suffer from gastrointestinal conditions. Ln, several instances many patients say, "The doctor told me my lab tests are standard and my pancreas is okay.

"Not to be the carrier of immoral news, though many lab tests are done these days in medical facilities are regular non-specific tests. These tests may not be looking for the indicators that point to a low-functioning pancreas.

If a person is in the commencement stages of chronic pancreatitis, that person cannot depend on standard, nondescript tests to save the day. Rather than putting your faith in incomplete blood tests, the symptoms that a person is experiencing will assist a medical professional.

Abdominal pain and bloating, gas, constipation, diarrhea, and heartburn are saying something and offering valuable clues. By concentrating on the symptoms, a medical practitioner can assist a person's pancreas to get the help that it desires.
It has been scientifically established that acidity destroys the pancreas.

One medical article, "Chronic Metabolic Acidosis Destroys Pancreas" in the European Journal of Pancreas, discusses this cause and effect situation. Good news!
In this case, you do not require a fancy test. You alone can check your body's acidity by putting your saliva and urine on litmus paper.

You are testing to see what the pH of your saliva and urine are. If their pH is less than 6.6, you have full body acidity.

If your saliva and urine are acidic, less than 6.6 pH, your bile and the pancreatic juice are also acidic. The Translation-your pancreas is weak and needs support; it is not functioning optimally.

Millions of Americans suffer from functional disorders of the gastrointestinal (G.I.) tract, like functional dyspepsia, irritable bowel syndrome (IBS), gastroesophageal reflux disease (GERD), bile dyskinesia, constipation, etc.

These illnesses are mentioned as functional disorders since the body is not correctly digesting food; this bodily function is lessened in some way. Typically, these functional disorders do not include structural harm to the G.I. tract.

With most of these functional disorders, the pancreas is not functioning as it should since mild chronic pancreatitis exists.

The way the human pancreas was fashioned, it has a 90% capacity. It shows that if only

10% or less of the pancreas is still working, then dangerous, life-threatening symptoms can appear in the human being.

Moreover, the pancreas seldom loses 90% of its function overnight. Generally, it takes about9 -15 years to go from the first incidence of pancreatitis to the end-stage of chronic pancreatitis.

From the beginning, it is time to take action!

Regrettably, modern medicine habitually kicks into gear too late in the game. When a patient has gotten to the end stage, there is not much transformative work that can be done. With only 10% of the pancreas functioning, the end stage of pancreatitis is life-threatening.

Is there a way to help the pancreas recuperate that does not need drugs or surgery? As the proverbial drum rolls, the answer is yes! The pancreas agonizes because its core has been dented. What is the pancreas' core? Pancreatic juice is at the center of the pancreas.

If pancreatic juice shorts of water, minerals, trace elements, bicarbonate, and proteins, moreover, it cannot function well. You can't get water from a dry well!

To reload the pancreas with the water, minerals, trace elements, and bicarbonate that it requires, many have switched to Karlovy Vary's healing mineral water.

In Europe, there is a healing spring in a small town in the Czech Republic called Karlovy Vary or "Carlsbad" in English. For over 520 years, European doctors have been recommending Karlovy Vary's healing mineral water to treat digestive disorders.

What the pancreatic juice is missing, this healing mineral water has. It has the minerals, trace elements, and bicarbonate that the pancreas genuinely requires. The surprising make-up of this healing water is fundamental to its healing power.

As Karlovy Vary healing mineral water has existed for a long time, many studies and tests have been done on it by the European medical sector.

According to European doctors, this healing water increases the quantity of pancreatic juice formed, and the quality of the pancreatic juice overall is better.

The Karlovy Vary healing mineral water also generates an alkaline environment in the small intestine. In an alkalized environment, pancreatic digestive enzymes can work appropriately.

Since Karlovy Vary mineral water has been around for at least 500 years, millions of persons historically have enhanced their health by drinking this healing water. In the beginning, individuals would travel to the Karlovy Vary spring to drink its healing water.

In 1765, this healing water was made portable. The healing water would evaporate into a salt form, which could be shipped to people.

Persons could get the healing water in its salt state, add water, drink it, and get the same healing that individuals were getting who went directly to the Karlovy Vary spring. So many persons who couldn't pay to travel to the Karlovy Vary healing spring or couldn't make the trip physically were getting better.

Proven and tested, Karlovy Vary healing mineral water assist 2 main pancreatic-related ailments-diabetes and chronic pancreatitis.

According to the latest data, there are about 90,000 new cases of pancreatitis yearly in the United States. The data also notes that 950,000 ambulatory care visits each year owing to pancreatitis.

These numbers only talk about the cases of pancreatitis that are reported. Many more examples of milder types of pancreatitis also happen each year. Nevertheless, these milder cases may not be stated.

Quite a bit of information has been offered in this section of the ebook. **The main takeaways for the reader are:**

1. If somebody has a digestive disorder, their pancreatic function is not working optimally. Their pancreatic

juice and digestive enzymes are low quality and in low quantity. When the pancreas is deficient, the body can show one or more of the following symptoms--belching, heartburn, abdominal cramps and pain, nausea, bloating, diarrhea, gas, constipation, etc.

2. Pancreatic disorders with low pancreatic function are more pronounced than people may think. Some professionals revealed that 14% of all dead people had pancreatic problems.
They may or may not have acknowledged that they had the pancreatic disease; moreover, 12% of the annual deaths had some pancreatic illness level.

3. The earlier an individual gets treatment for a pancreatic disorder, the better! More profound healing can happen in the previous stages of pancreatic illness.

4. Non-drug, non-surgery healing approaches can improve a person's quality

of life and postpone or even eliminate the worsening of pancreatic disorders.
Alternative medicinal therapies can work with usual treatments. An individual does not need to pick just one therapy method, though you can use both alternative therapies and traditional pancreatic recovery methods.

5. Alternative medicine has been verified and proven to be successful in assisting people with pancreatic disorders. Some alternative medicinal methods consist of:
- Drinking Karlovy Vary healing mineral water
- Going for Acupuncture
- Following a curative alkalized diet
- Using herbs
- Using chiropractor and abdominal managements
- Eating nutritional supplements
- Participating in medical hypnosis and other methods of relaxation

6. Use a qualified, experienced specialist(s) who comprehends pancreatic disorders and which treatments work.

Chapter 10

Natural Remedies for Pancreatitis Relief

Pancreatitis is a harrowing condition marked by inflammation of the pancreas—a large gland that plays a strategic part in regulating digestion. Whereas chronic pancreatitis needs ongoing care, acute pancreatitis needs instant medical attention.

Many natural remedies (used to complement but not swap conventional care) may help ease pain and other pancreatitis symptoms for chronic patients.

Situated behind your stomach, the pancreas discharges enzymes into your small intestine to stimulate food breakdown. When pancreatitis happens, those enzymes wrongly attack the very tissues that produce them.

There are two kinds of pancreatitis: acute and chronic. The more common type is acute pancreatitis, a situation that accounts for about 280,000 hospital stays in the U.S. each year. Often triggered by gallstones, acute pancreatitis produces such symptoms as severe pain in the upper abdomen, nausea, and vomiting.

Treatment typically consists of hospital treatment with intravenous (IV) fluids, antibiotics, and pain medication.

The most common cause of chronic pancreatitis is heavy alcohol usage, with symptoms comprising nausea, vomiting, weight loss, and oily stools. Known to deteriorate over time, chronic pancreatitis can lead to permanent harm and lead to diabetes, kidney failure, and breathing problems.

To lessen your pancreatitis risk, it's imperative to restrict your alcohol intake. Sustaining a healthy weight, holding to a balanced eating plan, and getting ample exercise may also be suggested.

Pancreatitis and Your Diet:

Following a low-fat diet that restricts greasy, fried, and high-fat processed foods are frequently suggested for both averting and handling pancreatitis.

That's because overeating fat can cause your pancreas to discharge more digestive enzymes than it typically would.
An excessive level of enzymes may lead to an attack.
The National Pancreas Foundation counsels that patients with pancreatitis restrict their fat intake to 22 grams or fewer per day, with no one meal comprising more than 12 grams of Fat.
Drinking plenty of fluids and cutting back on caffeine is also proposed for people with pancreatitis, according to the National Institute of Diabetes and Digestive and Kidney Diseases.

In some cases of pancreatitis, patients may need to obtain total parenteral nutrition. A feeding process that circumvents the gastrointestinal tract, complete parenteral nutrition, offers the patient's daily requirement of nutrients by intravenous drip.

Healthy Foods to Eat With Chronic Pancreatitis:

Pancreatitis and Weight Loss

With acute pancreatitis becoming more common in the U.S., it's projected that the obesity epidemic may be a reason for rising rates of this disease. What's more, a study circulated in *Current Opinion in Gastroenterology* in 2019 shows that obesity may exacerbate the severity of acute pancreatitis.

For assistance in keeping your weight in check—and probably guarding against pancreatitis check out the remedies below.

Remedies for Pancreatitis Relief

Although research on the use of natural remedies for pancreatitis relief is restricted, there's some initial evidence that certain supplements may lessen symptoms. Here's a look at numerous findings from those studies:

Antioxidants

Antioxidants may somewhat lessen pain in people with chronic pancreatitis, according to a report distributed in *The Cochrane Database of Systematic Reviews* in 2018. For this report, scientists analyzed 14 previously published clinical trials with a total of 589 partakers.

In their conclusion, they noted that the "clinical significance of this small reduction is indefinite, and more confirmation is required." They also found that contrary events, while mostly mild, happened in 17percent of participants.5

It's believed that taking antioxidant supplements may help treat chronic pancreatitis by decreasing oxidative stress (a likely factor in the development of this disease). It should be noted that, in a systematic review published in 2015, researchers analyzed 24 clinical trials and established that the data do not support a benefit of antioxidant therapy in the management of pancreatitis.

Glutamine:

An amino acid undoubtedly present in your body, glutamine plays a part in many metabolic processes. Some research shows that glutamine supplementation may help people with acute pancreatitis who get total parenteral nutrition.

For a report published in the journal *Pancreatology* in 2018, researchers studied 14 clinical trials with a total of 507 patients. According to the report's authors, their analysis "validates a clear benefit" for glutamine supplementation in patients with acute pancreatitis getting total parenteral nutrition.

They also noted that those getting enteral nutrition (food supplied to the stomach or small intestine through a tube) do not need glutamine.7

Omega-3 Fatty Acids

The use of omega-3 fatty acids may help lessen infectious problems and length of hospital stay in folks with acute pancreatitis, above all, when used parenterally. That's the finding of a 2018 report issued in the journal *Nutrients*, which analyzed ten clinical trials.

A class of polyunsaturated fats and omega-3 fatty acids are naturally found in various foods (containing flaxseed and fatty fish like salmon and tuna). Initial research suggests that omega-3 fatty acids may help treat pancreatitis by decreasing inflammation and restoring tissue damage.

Should You Use Natural Remedies for Pancreatitis Relief?

Owing to a lack of large-scale medical trials testing their effects in the management of pancreatitis, it's too soon to propose any natural remedies for pancreatitis relief. If you're excited about using natural remedies to manage pancreatitis pain, talk to your consultant first about how to incorporate such remedies into your treatment plan.

Keep in mind that acute pancreatitis could be life-threatening. If you experience symptoms such as severe pain that begins gradually or unexpectedly in your upper abdomen, look for medical help right away.

Natural Relief from Pancreatitis Pain

The pancreas is a large organ positioned in the abdomen that controls the production and discharge of enzymes that assist in the digestive processes. It is also in control of the production of Insulin and glucagon, the two hormones that control blood sugar.

Pancreatic disorders can result in inflammation of the organ, and an over secretion of hyper-activated enzymes.

These enzymes, so needed for digestion and the absorption of nutrients, start to attack the neighboring tissue repeatedly, causing acute and chronic pain. The most common symptoms connected with pancreatitis are abdominal pain, swelling of the abdomen, nausea, and a quickening pulse.

Those suffering through bouts of pancreatitis know just how agonizing and intrusive these attacks can be, though with natural therapies they can soon get relief the relief they seek for

Pancreatic Pain Relief the Natural Way:

One of the essential ways to help relieve pancreatitis is to consume raw, blended plant food with digestive enzymes.

This significantly cuts the work the pancreas has to do to digest food. In principle, it provides the pancreas a time of rest, which is considerably required to rebuild it.

Many patients suffering from pancreatitis have gotten relief from their symptoms through the therapeutic use of natural herbal supplements.

These herbal remedies, along with alternative treatments, have long been of help in ancient times up to these days.

Herbs such as milk thistle, red clover, and garlic have been used over the centuries to offer much-desired relief from the pain and inflammation triggered by pancreatitis.

Burdock root is always used to stimulate and sustain the overall health of the pancreas. At the same time, dandelion is mainly effective in cleansing the liver and bloodstream of toxins that can contribute to pancreatitis' chronic symptoms.

The use of more normally known dietary supplements, like selenium and beta carotene, also is confirmed useful in the treatment of pancreatitis.

These supplements, along with vitamins C, B3 and B5, contain, potent antioxidants like glutathione, CoQ10, and alpha-lipoic acid to sustain the health of the pancreas, while combating free radicals that can harm the organ. Those suffering from disorders of the pancreas are also advised to add vitamin E in the form of sunflower seeds to their daily regimen.

Vitamin E is critical to sustaining the health of all of the body's organs and can

help reverse the tissue destruction caused by chronic pancreatitis.

Alternative Physical Therapies for Pancreatitis

In addition to a daily routine of vitamin and herbal supplements, there are some alternative physical therapies and alternative treatments that relieve the symptoms of pancreatitis.

Pulsed electromagnetic field therapy is useful when the pancreas is swollen, as is bio photon cold laser treatments.

Colon hydrotherapy and lymphatic drainage therapy help lessen the toxic load, which helps the pancreas to rebuild.

Prayer and meditation on God's word can also be significantly effective in helping patients sustain the chronic symptoms of pancreatitis. Even though the blend of

breathing exercises and mental discipline, patients learn to manage their pain short

of the use of drugs or chemicals.

Prayer and meditation on God's word concentrating on the complete wholeness of body, mind, and spirit can have a common healing effect on the body.

Prayer and meditation on God's word decrease mental and physical stress, freeing the body from starting the healing process.

Pancreatitis can frequently lead to other more severe health conditions, comprising diabetes, malnutrition, kidney disorders, and pancreatic cancer.

Patients suffering from this ailment should speak with their holistic clinicians to design an appropriate treatment program.

Natural therapies can do more than simply lessen the symptoms of pancreatitis; they can assist the body restore much of the harm that has already been done.

Through a complete therapy schedule, people suffering from pancreatitis can find the relief they sort from their excruciating symptoms and take their first steps on the path to renewed health and vigor.

Chapter 11

Pancreatitis Diet:

CHRONIC PANCREATITIS PAIN MANAGEMENT AND TREATMENT

Pain Management

Substantial pain related to chronic pancreatitis can undermine a patient's quality of life. It is imperative to treat chronic pancreatitis as soon as it is diagnosed because frequent episodes of inflammation can cause irreparable damage, and pain relief becomes much less effective.

Pain relief can be attained with medication, often using the World Health Organization's 3-step ladder method to pain relief:

1 Pain medication commences with no opioids (such as acetaminophen, ibuprofen, or both).

2. If nonopioids do not ease pain, slight opioids (like codeine) are specified.
3. If minor opioids do not relieve pain, potent opioids (like morphine) are given.

Many patients with chronic pancreatitis get antioxidants with their pain medicine, which has been shown to assist with pain relief.3-5 There are other choices for pain relief, such as a celiac plexus block, which may offer another option for substantial pain relief.

The celiac plexus block is attained through injection and averts the nerves that travel from the pancreas from reporting pain signals back to the brain.
If there is a constricting of the pancreatic duct, placement of a plastic tube termed a stent into the duct can be helpful in lessening pain symptoms.

Restricted Role of Endoscopic Retrograde Cholangiopancreatography (ERCP)
An ERCP test, in which a flexible endoscope is positioned into the intestine, and a catheter is used to inject dye into the pancreas, should typically not be used in chronic pancreatitis, and it should never be used to treat chronic pancreatitis because injecting dye into the pancreas can lead to pancreatitis.

Surgery:

When medical therapy fails to offer relief to patients with chronic pancreatitis, surgical therapy may be a choice. A lateral pancreatojejunostomy (improved Puestow procedure) can result in pain relief in up to 83% of patients.

Whipple Procedure:

Another surgical procedure, which can eradicate inflammation and masses on the head of the pancreas, is the standard Whipple procedure; moreover, this practice does get rid of a lot of vital tissue and can be linked with complications such as the increased risk of death.

When possible, reformed Whipple procedures are done to save more tissue likened to the classic Whipple procedure, and can be useful for pain relief and return to daily activity.

TPIAT:

For suitably selected patients whose pain remains debilitating despite standard medical and surgical methods, total pancreatectomy with islet autotransplantation (TP-IAT) – while not a panacea – produces substantial relief of symptoms...

Antioxidant therapies:

Basic and clinical evidence proposes that the development of both acute pancreatitis (A.P.) and chronic pancreatitis (C.P.) can be linked with oxidative stress. Discoveries show that free radical activity and oxidative stress indices are higher in the blood and duodenal juice of patients with pancreatitis.

Based on these discoveries, the idea of using antioxidant regimens in the management of both A.P. and C.P. as a supplement and complementary in combination with its traditional therapy is sensible. In practice, moreover, the complete effectiveness of antioxidants is not recognized, and the best mixture of agents and dosages is not clear. Presently, a trial of a combination of antioxidants comprising vitamin C, vitamin E, selenium, and methionine is rational as one element of overall medical management.

In summary, there is no definite agreement on the dosage, length of therapy, and, eventually, the advantages of antioxidant therapy in the management of A.P. or C.P. Moreover, well-designed clinical studies are required to determine the suitable combination of agents, time of initiation, and period of therapy.

Bilateral Thoracoscopic Splanchnicectomy:

This is a choice for intractable chronic pain, but it is not extensively available. It is surgical resection of one or more of the splanchnic nerves for the handling of intractable pain. It is typically performed by a thoracic surgeon when it is done.

The following treatments are usually suggested for chronic pancreatitis.

Lifestyle changes. Folks with **chronic pancreatitis** will need to undertake some lifestyle changes. Bring to an end alcohol consumption and tobacco use.
·Pain management.

Treatment should not only concentrate on helping ease the pain symptoms but moreover also depression, which is a typical result of long-term pain.
·**Insulin.** The pancreas may stop manufacturing Insulin if the harm is extensive. The individual is likely to have developed diabetes type 1. Regular insulin treatment will become part of the handling for the rest of the person's life

Endoscopic surgery. A narrow, hollow, flexible tube named an endoscope is implanted into the digestive system, conducted by ultrasound. A device with a tiny, flattened balloon at the end is threaded through the endoscope. When it gets the duct, the balloon is inflated, hence widening the duct. A stent is positioned to stop the duct from constricting back.

Pancreas resection. (1) **The Beger method:** This contains resection of the swollen pancreatic head with cautious sparing of the duodenum; the rest of the pancreas is rewired to the intestines.

The Frey procedure: This is used when the doctor believes pain is triggered by inflammation of the head of the pancreas and the blocked ducts. The Frey procedure adds a longitudinal duct decompression to the pancreatic head resection - the head of the pancreas is surgically eliminated.

The ducts are decompressed by linking them directly to the intestines. (3) **Pylorus-sparing pancreaticoduodenectomy (PPPD):** The gallbladder, ducts, and the head of the pancreas are all surgically detached.

Total pancreatectomy. This consist of the surgical eradication of the whole pancreas

Autologous pancreatic islet cell transplantation (APICT).

During the total pancreatectomy process, a suspension of secluded islet cells is generated from the surgically removed pancreas and injected into the liver's portal vein. The islets cells will function as a free graft in the liver and will produce Insulin.

Chapter 12

7-Day Pancreatitis Diet Meal Plan

Pancreatitis arises when the pancreas that produces your digestive enzymes becomes swollen.

The pancreas yields Insulin and digestive enzymes, though these enzymes may end irritating the organ itself. This irritation may halt the pancreas from carrying out its function, and this condition is termed pancreatitis.

Because of the close nature of the pancreas and the digestive system, what you select to eat can have a primary effect.

Although gallstones habitually cause pancreatitis inflammation, chronic pancreatitis is even more carefully connected to your day-to-day diet.

This part of the ebook will cover everything you ought to know about following a diet to help with pancreatitis and give a sample 7-day plan to follow.

Pancreatitis Diet Foods to Eat

Furthermore, a pancreas-friendly diet comprises lots of Protein from lean meats and little animal fat or simple sugar.
This means you should get the bulk of your protein sources from poultry, seafood, and low-fat dairy.
If you eat red meats, make sure you get lean meats with condensed saturated Fat.
These foods should make up the bulk of your meals:

- **Dairy** – low-fat cheeses such as feta and mozzarella, low-fat milk and yogurt, eggs
- **Fruits and vegetables** – all types of fruit and veg. Higher fat fruits and

vegetables such as avocado are sufficient in moderation.

- **Beans and legumes** – black beans, chickpeas, lentils
- **Whole grains** – whole grain bread with pasta, barley, brown rice, oats, quinoa

Chronic pancreatitis can usually cause malnutrition as the pancreas doesn't function efficiently. You should be conscious that Vitamins A, D, E, and K are most commonly found to be missing due to pancreatitis.

Vitamin deficiency owing to malabsorption can cause osteoporosis, digestive problems, and other warning sign.

Pancreatitis Diet Foods to Shun

These are the types of foods you should limit or circumvent:

Organ meats – liver, kidneys, heart

Fried foods – French fries, donuts, and fried meats are extraordinary in saturated fats

Treated meats – sausages and bacon

Drinks with added sugar – fruit juices and soda

Alcohol – alcohol intake can exacerbate a pancreatitis attack acute and add to chronic pancreatitis

Full-fat dairy – high-fat cheese (e.g., cheddar and brie) and whole milk has a lot of saturated Fat

High-fat spreads – margarine and butter

To be specific, cooked or deep-fried foods may cause a pancreatitis flare-up. Refined grains such as white bread, flour, and rice can also be challenging as they cause your insulin levels to spike.

Alcohol can also aggravate an acute pancreatitis attack and contribute to chronic pancreatitis. Many of us <u>drink too much</u> already, and substantial alcohol intake has been linked with increased pancreatic cancer risk.

Selecting a Pancreatitis Diet:

Some investigation says that some people can tolerate approximately 32-43% of their calories from fat when it's from whole-food plant sources or medium-chain triglycerides (MCT).

Others may find that they work better with less fat in their diet, though you'll typically want a **medium fat diet that's majorly plant-based and low in saturated fats.**

The Mediterranean diet fits this description well.
It centers on the foods mentioned above and prioritizes fats from healthy sources like extra virgin olive oil rather than saturated fats.

Many leading organizations back eating a Mediterranean diet for pancreatitis as well as whole health, comprising:
- Harvard Medical School
- Cleveland Clinic
- Arthritis Foundation
- Mayo Clinic

It also reliably tops the best diets to follow because of how healthy it is and how viable it is to follow over the long-term. U.S. News ranked it as the number 1 diet.

This is great for folks who want a long-term answer that they can stick to forever rather than a short-term fix.

Several studies have shown that the Mediterranean diet can assist with a collection of health-related diseases, like:

· Reduced threat of cardiovascular events, coronary heart disease,
· Reduced Danger of coronary heart disease
· Reduced risk of getting type 2 diabetes
· Danger of breast cancer
· Reduced obesity
· Improved cognitive function

Pancreatitis Diet Meal Plan
Pancreatitis Diet Sample Menu
In this meal plan are recipes for breakfast, lunch, and dinner.

Breakfast
Lunch
Dinner

Monday

Banana Yogurt Pots
Cannellini Bean Salad
Swift Moussaka

Tuesday

Tomato with Watermelon Salad
Edgy Veggie Wraps
Peppery Tomato Baked Eggs

Wednesday

Blueberry Oats Bowl
Fresh Carrot, with Orange and Avocado Salad
Fresh Salmon with Potatoes and Corn Salad

Thursday

Banana Yogurt Pots
Assorted Bean Salad
Flavored Carrot and Lentil Soup

Friday

Tomato with Watermelon Salad
Panzanella with fresh Salad
Med Chicken, Quinoa, and Swiss Salad

Saturday

Blueberry Oats Dish
Quinoa and Stir Cooked Veg
Sautéed Vegetables with Bean Mash

Sunday

Banana Yogurt Pans
Algerian Chickpea Soup
Highly spiced Mediterranean Beet Salad

Snacks are suggested between mealtimes. Some tasty snacks comprise:
· A handful of nuts or seeds
· A bit of fruit
· Carrots or baby carrots
· Berries, grapes , avocado

- **Day 1: Monday**

Breakfast: Banana Yogurt Pots

Nutrition

- Calories – 238
- Protein – 15g
- Carbs – 34g
- Fat – 8g

Prep time: 7 minutes

Ingredients (for 2 persons)
- 227g Greek yogurt
- 3 bananas, cut up into chunks
- 17g walnuts, toasted and chopped

Instructions

1. Put some of the yogurts into the bottom of a glass. Complement a layer of banana, after yogurt and repeat. As soon as the glass is full, scatter with the nuts.

Lunch: Cannellini Bean Salad

Nutrition
- Calories – 303
- Protein – 24g
- Carbs – 56g
- Fat – 0g

Prep time: 6 minutes

Ingredients (for 2 persons)

- 610g cans cannellini beans
- 72g cherry tomatoes halved
- ½ red onion, finely divided
- ½ tbsp red wine vinegar
- small bunch basil, torn

Instructions

1. Wash and drain the beans and blend with the tomatoes, onion, and vinegar. Season, then supplement basil just before serving.

Dinner: Quick' n'Easy Moussaka

Nutrition
- Calories – 576
- Protein – 28g
- Carbs – 47g
- Fat – 28g

Prep time + Cook time: 32 minutes

Ingredients (for 3 persons)
- 1 tbsp additional virgin olive oil
- ½ onion, superbly cut
- 1 garlic clove, wonderfully sliced
- 253g lean beef mince
- 220g can cut tomatoes
- 1 tbsp tomato purée
- 1 tsp crushed cinnamon
- 220g can chickpeas
- 105g pack feta cheese smashed
- Mint (fresh desirable)
- Brown bread, to serve

Instructions

1. Heat the oil in a saucepan. Add the onion and garlic and stir fry till soft. Add the mince and fry for 3-5 minutes until grilled.
2. Put the tomatoes into the pot and combination in the tomato purée and cinnamon, then season. Allow the mince to seethe for 22 minutes. Add the chickpeas midway through.
3. Peppering the feta and mint over the mince. Serve with grilled bread.

Day 2: Tuesday

Breakfast: Tomato and Watermelon Salad

Nutrition
· Calories – 178
· Protein – 7g
· Carbs – 16 g

· Fat – 14g
Prep time + Cook time: 7 minutes
Ingredients (for 3 persons)
· 2 tbsp olive oil
· 2 tbsp red wine vinegar
· ¼ tsp chill flakes

- 1 tbsp sliced mint
- 122g tomatoes, sliced
- 255g watermelon, cut into pieces
- 53g feta cheese, crushed

Instructions

1. For the dressing, mix the oil, vinegar, chili flakes, and mint and then season.
2. Put the tomatoes and watermelon into a bowl. Pour over the dressing, add the feta, then serve.

Lunch: Edgy Veggie Wraps

Nutrition
- Calories – 320
- Protein – 13g
- Carbs – 41g
- Fat – 12g

Prep time + Cook time: 12 minutes

Ingredients (for 3 folks)
- 110g cherry tomatoes
- 2 cucumbers
- 7 Kalamata olives
- 2 sizeable wholemeal tortilla wraps
- 52g feta cheese
- 2 tbsp houmous

Instructions

1. Cut the tomatoes, slice the cucumber into sticks, divide the olives and take out the stones.
2. Heat the tortillas.

3. Spread the houmous over the wrap. Place the vegetable mixture in the middle and roll-up.

Dinner: Spicy Tomato Baked Eggs
Nutrition
· Calories – 418
· Protein – 20g
· Carbs – 46g
· Fat – 19g

Prep time + Cook time: 27 minutes

Ingredients (for 3 persons)
· 2 tbsp olive oil
· 2 red onions, sliced
· 1 red chili, pitted & sliced
· 1 garlic clove, divided
· small bunch coriander stalks and leaves sliced separately
· 803g can cherry tomatoes
· 5 eggs
· brown bread, to serve

Instructions
1. Heat the oil in a frying pan with a lid, then boil the onions, chili, garlic and coriander stalks for 7 minutes till soft. Stir in the tomatoes, then cook for 9-12 minutes.
2. Using the back of a large spoon, make 5 dips in the sauce, then crack an egg into each one. Place a lid on the pan, then cook over low heat for 6-9 mins, until the eggs are

done to your taste. Sprinkle with the coriander leaves and serve with bread.

Day 3: Wednesday

Breakfast: Blueberry Oats Dish

Nutrition

· Calories – 236
· Protein – 14g
· Carbs – 39g
· Fat – 5g

Prep time + Cook time: 12 minutes
Ingredients (for 3 persons)
· 62g porridge oats
· 170g French yogurt
· 176g blueberries
· 1 tsp honey

Instructions
1. Placed the oats in a saucepan with 405ml of water. Heat and stir for about 3 minutes. Take away from the heat and add a third of the yogurt.
2. Tip the blueberries into a saucepan with the honey and 1 tbsp of water. Lightly poach until the blueberries are gentle.

3. Spoon the porridge into plates and add the leftover yogurt and blueberries.

Lunch: Carrot, Orange and Avocado Salad

Nutrition
· Calories – 178
· Protein – 6g
· Carbs – 15g
· Fat – 15g

Prep time + Cook time: 7 minutes

Ingredients (for 3 folks)
· 1 orange, and more zest and juice of 1
· 2 carrots, halved along the length and cut up with a peeler
· 36g bag rocket/arugula
· 1 avocado, stoned, skinned and cut up
· 1 tbsp olive oil

Instructions
1. Cut the sections from 1 of the oranges and put in a basin with the carrots, rocket, and avocado. Stick together the orange juice, zest, and oil. Toss through the Salad, and season it.

Dinner: Salmon sandwiched with Potatoes and Corn Salad

Nutrition
· Calories – 480
· Protein – 45g
· Carbs – 28g

- Fat – 22g

Prep time + Cook time: 32 minutes

Ingredients (for 3 persons)
- 210g baby new potatoes
- 1 sweetcorn cob
- 2 skinless salmon bones
- 70g tomatoes
- 1 tbsp red wine vinegar
- 1 tbsp extra-virgin olive oil
- 1 shallot, superbly cut
- 1 tbsp capers, excellently severed
- handful basil leaves

Instructions

1. Cook potatoes in boiling water up until it is soft, adding corn for the last 6 minutes. Drain & cool.
2. For the dressing, blend the vinegar, oil, shallot, capers, basil & flavor.
3. Heat grill to high. Brush some dressing on salmon & cook, peeled side down, for 7-9 minutes. Cut tomatoes & place them on the plate. Cut the potatoes, cut the corn from the cob & add to plate. Add the salmon & sprinkle over the remaining dressing.

Day 4: Thursday

Breakfast: Banana Yogurt Vessels

Lunch: Blend Bean Salad

Nutrition
· Calories – 243
· Protein – 12g
· Carbs – 23g
· Fat – 13g

Prep time + Cook time: 12 minutes
Ingredients (for 3 folks)
· 146g jar artichoke heart in oil
· ½ tbsp. well-preserved tomato paste
· ½ tsp red wine vinegar
· 210g can cannellini beans, drained and washed
· 155g pack tomatoes, subdivided handful Kalamata black olives
· 2 spring onions, thinly cut up on the diagonal
· 110g feta cheese pounded

Instructions
1. Trench the jar of artichokes, keeping 1-2 tbsp of oil. Add the oil, sun-dried tomato paste, and vinegar and mix until smooth. Season to taste.

2. Slice the artichokes and tip into a dish. Add the cannellini beans, tomatoes, olives, spring onions, and half of the feta cheese. Mix in the artichoke oil blend and tip into a serving bowl. Smash over the outstanding feta cheese, then serve.

Dinner: Flavored Carrot and Lentil Soup
Nutrition
· Calories – 239
· Protein – 12g
· Carbs – 35g
· Fat – 8g

Prep time + Cook time: 26 minutes
Ingredients (for 3 persons)
· 1 tsp cumin seeds
· pinch chili flakes
· 1 tbsp olive oil
· 310g carrots washed and rudely peeved (no need to peel)
· 72g split red lentils
· 505ml hot vegetable stock (from a cube is well)
· 62ml milk
· Greek yogurt, to serve

Instructions
1. Heat a big saucepan and dry fry the cumin seeds and chili flakes for 2 minutes. Scoop out about half of the seeds with a spoon and put aside. Add the oil, carrot, lentils, stock,

and milk to the saucepan and bring to the boil. Simmer for 17 minutes until the lentils have swollen and become softer.
2. Whizz the broth with a stick Whizzer or in a food mixer until smooth. Spice to taste and finish with a dollop of French yogurt and a bit of the reserved meshed spices.

Day 5: Friday

Breakfast: Tomato and Watermelon Salad

Lunch: Panzanella Salad

Nutrition
· Calories – 453
· Protein – 7g
· Carbs – 38g
· Fat – 26g
Prep time + Cook time: 12 minutes
Ingredients (for 3 persons)
· 410g tomatoes
· 1 garlic clove, crushed
· 1 tbsp capers, drained and dipped
· 1 suitable avocado, stoned, peeled and sliced
· 1 small red onion, very finely divided

- 2 pieces of brown bread
- 2 tbsp olive oil
- 1 tbsp red wine vinegar
- small handful basil leaves

Instructions

1. Cut the tomatoes and put them in a vessel. Flavor well and add the garlic, capers, avocado, and onion. Blend well and set aside for 10 minutes.

2. In the meantime, rip the bread into pieces and place in a bowl. Sprinkle over half of the olive oil and half of the vinegar. When ready to serve, strew tomatoes and basil leaves and sprinkle with left over oil and vinegar. Stir well /before serving.

Dinner: Med Chicken, Quinoa, and Greek Salad

Nutrition

- Calories – 474
- Protein – 37g
- Carbs – 58g
- Fat – 26g

Prep time + Cook time: 22 minutes

Ingredients (for 3 persons)

- 110g quinoa
- ½ red chili, deseeded and excellently sliced
- 1 garlic clove, crushed
- 205g chicken
- 1 tbsp extra-virgin olive oil

- 152g tomato, unevenly sliced
- handful pitted black Kalamata olives
- ½ red onion, wonderfully chopped
- 55g feta cheese smashed
- small bunch mint leaves, cut
- juice and zest ½ lemon

Instructions

1. Boil the quinoa following the pack instructions, then wash in cold water and drain carefully.
2. In the meantime, toss the chicken fillets in the olive oil with flavor, chili, and garlic. Put in a hot pan and boil for 3-5 minutes each side or till cooked through. Transfer it to a plate and set it aside
3. Next, tip the tomatoes, olives, onion, feta, and mint into a container. Toss in the boiled quinoa. Stir through the outstanding olive oil, lemon juice and zest, and season well. Serve with the chicken on top.

Day 6: Saturday

Breakfast: Blueberry Oats Bowl

Lunch: Quinoa and Blend Fried Veg

Nutrition
- Calories – 474
- Protein – 13g
- Carbs – 57g
- Fat – 26g

Prep time + Cook time: 32 minutes

Ingredients (for 3 persons)
- 130g quinoa
- 4 tbsp olive oil
- 2 garlic clove, excellently sliced
- 3 carrots, cut into thin sticks
- 155g leek cut up
- 153g broccoli, slice into small florets
- 55g tomatoes
- 120ml vegetable stock
- 1 tsp tomato paste
- juice ½ lemon

Instructions

1. Boil the quinoa according to pack instructions. In the meantime, heat 3 tbsp of the oil in a saucepan, then add the garlic and promptly fry for 2 minutes. Throw in the carrots, leeks, and <u>broccoli</u>, then stir-fry for 3 minutes until everything is sparkling.

2. Add the tomatoes, blend the stock and tomato paste, then add to the pan—cover and cook for 4 minutes. Drain the quinoa and toss in the leftover oil and lemon juice.

Divide between warm plates and spoon the vegetables on uppermost.

Dinner: Meshed Vegetables with Bean Mash

Nutrition
· Calories – 315
· Protein – 20g
· Carbs – 34g
· Fat – 17g

Prep time + Cook time: 42 minutes

Ingredients (for 3 persons)
· 1 tbsp olive oil
· 1 tbsp red wine vinegar
·
· 1/3 tsp chili flakes
· 1 tbsp sliced mint
· 123g tomatoes, sliced
· 255g watermelon, chopped into chunks
· 55g feta cheese, crushed

Instructions

1. Heat the grill. Organize the vegetables over a grill pan & brush carefully with oil. Grille until lightly browned, turn them over, brush again with oil, then grate until tender.

2. In the meantime, put the beans in a saucepan with garlic and stock. Bring to the simmer, then boil, open, for 11 minutes. Mash unevenly with a potato masher. Divide the vegetables and mash between 2 plates,

sprinkle over oil, and drizzle with black pepper and coriander.

Day 7: Sunday

Breakfast: Banana Yogurt Pots

Lunch: Moroccan Chickpea Broth

Nutrition

- Calories – 409
- Protein – 16g
- Carbs – 64g
- Fat – 12g

Prep time + Cook time: 27 minutes
Ingredients (for 3 folks)
- 1 tbsp olive oil
- ½ medium onion, sliced
- 1 celery sticks, cut
- 1 tsp ground cumin
- 305ml hot vegetable stock
- 200g can sliced tomatoes
- 200g can chickpeas, cleaned and drained
- 52g frozen broad beans
- zest and juice 1/3 lemon
- coriander & bread to serve

Instructions
1. Heat the oil in a pan and then stir fry the onion and celery for 12 minutes until it is well softened. Add the cumin and cook for an additional minute.
2. Put on the heat, then add the stock, tomatoes, chickpeas, and black pepper. Boil for 9 minutes. Add broad beans and lemon juice and cook for an additional 3 minutes. Top with lemon zest and coriander.

Dinner: Peppery Mediterranean Beet Salad
Nutrition
· Calories – 549
· Protein – 24g
· Carbs – 59g
· Fat – 21g

Prep time + Cook time: 42 minutes
Ingredients (for 3 persons)
· 9 fresh baby beetroots, or 4 medium, scrubbed
· ½ tbsp za'atar
· ½ tbsp sumac
· ½ tbsp ground cumin
· 410g can chickpeas, drained and washed
· 2 tbsp olive oil
· ½ tsp lemon zest
· ½ tsp lemon juice
· 210g Italian yogurt

- 1 tbsp harissa paste
- 1 tsp sliced red chili flakes
- mint leaves, cut, to serve

Instructions

1. Heat oven to 222C/200C fan/ gas 7. Halve or quarter beetroots depending on size. Blend spices together. On a huge baking tray, blend chickpeas and beetroot with the oil. Flavor it with salt & sprinkle over the flavors. Mix again. Heat for 32 minutes.

2. While the vegetables are cooking, blend the lemon zest and juice with the yogurt. Spin the harissa through and spread into a container. Top with the beetroot & chickpeas, and drizzle with the chili flakes & mint.

Pancreatitis Diet Shopping List

This shopping list agrees with the 7-day pancreatitis diet plan, serving 2 or more people. No snacks are incorporated.

Conclusion:

First of all, thank you for purchasing this book

Discover The Proven Methods To Eliminate Pancreatitis With This Superb Meal Plans In 30 Days

I know you could have picked any number of books to read, but you picked this book and for that I am extremely grateful.

I hope that it added at value and quality to your everyday life. If so, it would be really nice if you could share this book with your friends and family by posting to Facebook and Twitter.

If you enjoyed this book and found some benefit in reading this, I'd like to hear from you and hope that you could take some time to post a review on Amazon. Your feedback and support will help this author to greatly improve his writing craft for future projects and make this book even better

Conclusion:

www.ingramcontent.com/pod-product-compliance
Ingram Content Group UK Ltd.
Pitfield, Milton Keynes, MK11 3LW, UK
UKHW020704160725
6916UKWH00019B/216